Enduring Fountain

Rosemary Argente

First edition 2017
Second edition 2017

Cover: Photo by Donna Karim

ISBN: 978-0-9557327-2-0

Publishers: Asaina Books
Website: asainabooks.co.uk
Email: rosa@asainabooks.co.uk

Books by the same author:

Blantyre and Yawo Women
The Veil
The Promised Land – Companion to The Veil
Praying Mantis
Broken Temple
Praying Mantis
Difference
Share the Ride
Home From Home
Essays and Poetry
The Place Beyond
Caesar and Mapanga Homestead

Novels:
All Mine to Have
Farewell Sophomore
The Stream of Memory
A British Throne Scandal

Science Fiction:
Farewell to the Aeroplane

Booklets:
Journey of Discovery
Enduring Fountain – Health and Well-being
Katherine of the Wheel
Cooking With Asaina

ACKNOWLEDGMENTS

Thanks to Pam Hunter and Lorna Argente for their constructive criticism. Magdalena Staniszewska for a critical sampling of the recipes. Donna Karim for her help on Information Technology. Also thanks to the many persons who have contributed to the compilation of this booklet and a special "Thank you" to Lorna and Archie for organising a memorable Eightieth Birthday get-together in 2010. Also to Ian Upton, David Duddle, Mark Sherman and Brian Sherman for their invaluable help on computer technology.

The source on some of the information on herbal healing in this booklet, came from author's two grandmothers, who were both herbalist healers:

Asaina – 1884-1972: maternal, Malawi, Africa; and

Fatima –1872-1965:paternal, Mozambique, Africa, whose husband's grandfather (author's great, grandfather) left Jamnagar, India (Pakistan, since partition of India and Pakistani in 1947) in 1756 for Beira, Mozambique

FOREWORD

Samuel V Bhima

F.R.C.O.G.

This readable booklet has been written with the needs of many in mind, particularly for women as they advance in age. As life expectancy of women in the Western world is rising, it is desirable that the ageing process should be as untraumatic and fulfilling as possible. Without undesirable effects of a poor diet a changing physical appearance and lack of physical and mental activity.

Having known the author for over 60 years, and been impressed by her continuing youthfulness and good health in her ageing years, the advice and guidance she has included in this booklet can be helpful to anyone who is keen to maintain their vitality. The author was raised with an awareness of good health, not from a medical background but from practical basis given that medical treatment was not easily accessible in Sub-Saharan Africa. The 'self help' approach could be said to be in vogue in Britain today and in this concise and practical manual, the author has brought together the experience she has with careful research to the benefit of its readers.

The scope of the booklet is ambitious and the reader is guided through a process of self-discipline with rewarding results due to sensible eating and exercise. The breadth and the tips of advice that is provided in this self-help book is broad, and as a medical man I would be cautious in advising anyone to believe that what benefits another would benefit oneself. That said, many of the details that the author has shared (from motivation of care) are common sense approaches, worth trying if you are seeking an improvement in your general well being.

Lifestyle

Food is sustenance.
Eat to live, live not to eat.
Enough is as good as a feast.
Moderate eating,
Buys quality, not quantity.
In advancing age eat less,
But exercise not less.

Respect the sanctity of your body,

We are:
What we eat.

What we drink.

What we think.

What we do.

PROLOGUE

Caveat Emptor

This booklet contains tips based on things that have worked for the author personally after decades of trial and error. It should be noted that there is no supporting evidence for the remedies in this book that have worked for other people. Though the author wishes to share this information with those who may be interested, it is essential that the reader must first check with personal medical practitioner before following any of the tips. That "one man's food is poison for another" cannot be over-emphasised.

THE FIRST ALLIES

Water – is one of the first allies and the most healing element.

Our bodies are largely made up of water and varies according to gender. The amount of water in the human body ranges from 50-75%; and percentage in infants is much higher, around 75-78% water, dropping to 65% by one year of age. Water for the body is a 'home from home' panacea, and it can also be a natural detox – see below.

It is better to drink tap water than to drink bottled water in plastic containers - also consider the environmental litter aspect in all we do and be as close to nature as possible. But having said that, tap water contains chemicals intended to purify the water, therefore it is not best to drink water directly from the tap. First put tap water in a water filter and after 24 hours the chemicals will have evaporated. The filtered water may be used to boil for tea or any other use that requires hot water. The filtered water may be placed in glass bottles, not plastic, and stored in the fridge.

For most of the over sixties (for some well below this age) there may be a tendency to incontinence in varying degrees. Take water and fluids sensibly. Your daily water intake should be at least four to six glasses when you are at home and stop drinking by 5:00 pm for a good undisturbed night's rest. Before your outing and when away from home avoid drinking any water or *fluids,* to avoid discomfort (or accidents!).

Drink hot water – not warm - after every meal, to help the digestion system to melt fat and eliminate heartburn or indigestion. At other times drink plenty of filtered cold water but do not overdo it.

Relaxation – is as essential as exercise. Synchronisation of mind and body is central to our being for inner development and self-refinement, spiritual uplifting and balance.

This exercise may take 15 to 20 minutes: Ambience – a quiet-softly lit room with music playing a relaxing melody.

(There are many on the market to choose from.)

Sit in a comfortable arm-chair. Hands relaxed on your lap, stare eye-level at a point straight in front of you and close your eyes. Deep breathe in through the nose, hold and gently breathe out through the mouth. Relax whole body while counting backwards from 200 continue to relax upwards from feet, calves, thighs, buttocks, abdomen, chest, hands, arms, shoulders, neck, face, eyelids – you will become heavier and heavier. In deepening tranquillity form a picture into the abyss. My picture: sitting in a canoe pushed by invisible oars and sailing gently through an underground stream, flanked by green foliage and weeping willows of pale green. When you have counted 200, close your eyes and continue to relax for 5/10 minutes. Then count 1 to 5 and come out of the abyss. After this exercise your mind and body will be completely rejuvenated and relaxed. Aim to do this exercise at least twice a month.

Euphoria

At least twice a month *walk* to the top of a hill (we cannot all be mountain climbers!) or some apex nearest your home and find a spot surrounded by trees and foliage with a panoramic view. Once there, you will be exhilarated and euphoria will follow;

for you become part of the universe in a holistic sense. Euphoria is the reward for the effort of walking up to the apex which will give you the benefit of general physical and mental well-being.

Health and Remedies

Medical help

If you are ill seek medical help through conventional medicine and follow your general practitioner's advice and if so advised succumb to the surgeon's scalpel for parts of the body that can no longer function. The body is made up of trillions of different cells and some cells die before the body's clinical death. You will forever be indebted to the surgeons, doctors, nurses and physiotherapists – for they perform miracles – you become less physically challenged when you have received their help. Should you choose 'vanity surgery', face lifts, etc., just remember that the treated parts of your body will age faster than the rest of your body because of the interference with natural cells.

What to do should you get a heart attack:

Take a deep breath

Cough repeatedly, deep prolonged coughs, as if producing sputum from deep inside the chest. Repeat every 2 seconds without letting up until help arrives or heart beat is normal.

The deep breaths bring oxygen into the lungs.The coughs squeezes the heart, keep blood circulating and help to regain normal breathing till help comes or get to the hospital.

Source: Journal of the General Hospital, Rochester.

To help keep open the arteries of your heart take long brisk walks. In addition, do an indoor jumping exercise: jump on one spot at least for a minute – this exercise can be very tiring hence 1 minute at a time, or as many minutes as you can take up to 5. The secret is to tire yourself but not to the extent of not being able to talk. You may wish to alternate with rope skipping up to 50 skips or more depending on how you feel.

Burns:

Egg white for burns: cover the whole affected area with egg white. Once the egg dries out the burn and pain will disappear like magic! If it is a serious burn, do not repeat the egg white emergency treatment, seek medical help.

Cancer – prevention for cure:

Be aware of but do not shun alternative medicine to cure cancer. The best way to avoid diseases is by prevention as a way of life, or a lifestyle to follow. 'Prevention for Cure' means tackle cancer or any disease at the root: we are largely what we eat, drink, think and do. A positive attitude will conquer cancer. Any disease will feed on certain foods and fluids while other foods or fluids may disarm the disease. Though it is said: *"One man's meat is another man's poison."* The following are excerpts taken from my research on cancer.

Useful information:

1.Message from Rick Cantrell, PhD, MD, PsyD:

Email: rick.cantrell@live.com

2. Manioc's [cassava] Vitamin B17 kills the cancer cell in humans

Apricot seed kernels are used in the fight against cancer. The kernels contain Vitamin B17, and Vitamin B17 is used in medication to counter cancer. B17 tablets with apricot seed extract are available in Australia and in the US. All the information you need is available on the

www.worldwithoutcancer.com website.

This letter is about how manioc, which also contains Vitamin B17, has the potential to combat cancer.

3. From: Miriam Desanker <mjdesanker@yahoo.com>

To: undisclosed recipient <mjdesanker@yahoo.com>

Sent: Wed, March 9, 2011 6:00:51 PM

Subject: Fw: Fwd: FW: LEMONS are 10 000 times STRONGER than CHEMOTHERAPY ...

--- On Wed, 3/9/11, Nkhono Edna <ednankhono@yahoo.com> wrote: Fwd: FW: LEMONS are 10 000 times STRONGER than CHEMOTHERAPY ...InboxX

Cut Some Lemons Up – Let the kids suck On Them – Put a slice In Your Water glass etc . . .*USE as A Prevention . . .*

****

4. MacMillan

The following websites make diet recommendations: http://www.macmillan.org.uk/information-and-support/coping/maintaining-a-healthy-lifestyle/healthy-eating/how-to-maintain-a-healthy- diet.html

https://www.cancer.gov/publications/patient-education/eatinghints.pdfhttp://www.webmd.com/cancer/features/eating-treatmenthttp://www.canceractive.com/cancer-active-page-link.aspx?n=531

ALLIES	FOES
Water: Drink filtered water	Tap water not directly from the tap
Fresh fruit/vegetable juices	
Smoothies (liquidised fruit)	Water in plastic bottles.
Unsweetened soy milk	Fresh milk can cause mucus in
Green teas (preferably China)	some people, hence migraine;
There are different China teas	all food products made from milk.
decaffeinate tea	such as cheese, etc.
Use honey to sweeten drinks	Granulated sugar, sugar
or in cooking such as rice	substitutes and all artificial
Pudding, or use molasses.	sweeteners or substitutes.
Cassava contains Vitamim B17	Avoid salt that has been
which kills cancer cells in humans.	refined.
Decaffeinated coffee and tea.	

****

To keep osteoarthritis at bay

Method one:

1 teaspoon of nettle tea   )   make in individual strainer.

1 cup boiling water   )

Add 2 teaspoons of cider vinegar 1 teaspoon honey. Mix well and drink daily.

Method two:

Steam 4 clusters of broccoli and add one tablespoon of cider vinegar,

and serve as a vegetable.

Method three:

Daily or nightly take two teaspoons of honey mix in a small teaspoon of cinnamon powder.

Menopause:

Lifestyle and diet can improve the uncomfortable effects of the menopause. If you prefer not to take Hormone Replacement Tablets (HRT), there is a large selection of alternatives to HRT: particularly yams, cassava, sweet potatoes, agnus cactus, black chickpeas, cohosh, dandelion, dong, fresh fruit, hops, lentils, linseeds, oats, quai, red clover, rye, soya beans, soya milk and yoghurt, vegetables and whole grains.

Pelvic floor muscle exercises

Sit upright, or lie on your back with knees slightly apart. Lift the perineum, and squeeze the pelvic floor muscles, as if trying to stop the passage of urine at the front or trying to stop the passage of wind at the back and hold the squeeze for as long as you can. This exercise can be done any time anywhere: standing in a queue, waiting in the bank, for a bus, at the doctor's waiting room, or wherever, as a way of life.

Note: It would benefit man to refrain from asserting that this exercise is for women only - a healthy pelvis cannot be overemphasised for everyone as this also helps to avoid backache.

Teeth - daily and regular care:

Brush teeth, gently at all times lest you cause bleeding, with tooth paste of choice before breakfast. Choose a small toothbrush – the smaller the better, even child's toothbrush. Also use Inter-dental or Micro brushes for in-between the teeth. Brush again after breakfast with a sensitivity tooth paste and gargle with one teaspoon of honey and cinnamon powder mixed in hot water, and breath stays fresh throughout the day. Brush teeth after every meal, particularly after eating fish – fish is hard on the teeth – and before going to bed. At least once a week cleanse your mouth with a solution of half a teaspoon of salt in a glass of warm water. This is a cure for bleeding gums and strengthens the teeth.

Chewing salted cucumber also helps to keep mouth ulcers at bay. To strengthen and whiten teeth - peel and shred raw cassava and chew slowly.

Do not attempt to break cassava with your teeth you may be in danger of breaking a tooth!

Eat sugar cane to strengthen teeth and preserve energy. Do not be put off by the unladylike sucking noise from eating sugar cane. Sugar cane is available already cut into two inch squares in Asian shops, if you live in Europe. Get hold of one end, chew and suck the other end; turn it round, chew and such the other without putting the whole piece into your mouth.

On Beauty:

"There is no beauty on earth which exceeds the

natural loveliness of woman."   J Petit-Senn.

The following tips stay close to nature. The methods are simple, easy to follow and maintain. Beauty in a nutshell is a collection of good and healthy tips designed to become part of a lovely person. The tips will work if taken as a way of life, or adopted as an essential *part of your lifestyle.* Results should not be expected in a few weeks since the metabolism needs completely to absorb the chosen intake of food and fluid or exercises to show results – no item should be taken as a quick fix as it were a tablet to relieve a headache momentarily.

Face and Body: For a skin as soft as that of a baby do an out/inside treatment. <u>Externally:</u> Take a ripe avocado pear scoop out 2 teaspoons and mix with half a teaspoon of lemon juice. Apply and massage the mixture all over your face and rinse off with warm water. You may use the same mixture for your whole body using one half of ripe avocado and juice of half a lemon. Apply and massage the mixture all over your body. Shower off. <u>Internally:</u> Add avocado slices to your salad or eat them in the way you prefer.

Eyes: are mirrors of the soul and animated eyes speak volumes. Saturate two pieces of cotton wool in lukewarm water. Lie supine on the floor and place the cotton wool on each eyelid and completely relax; you will feel as if you rare suspended on the axis of the revolving earth. This is excellent particularly for tired eyes.

1. For eyesight improvement. Sit comfortably in an arm chair and pick a spot directly in front and focus on it. Begin with 3

minutes and increase to five minutes or more.

2. To strengthen your eyes: stand, or sit, erect with your arms at your sides and look straight ahead of you. Then only move your eyes clockwise: up to the ceiling; to the right; down to the floor; then to the left. Repeat five times then do the same anticlockwise. Apply a thin layer of castor oil to your eyes and eyebrows before going to bed. Do not do both 1 and 2 exercises at the same time; alternate in 24 hour intervals. This exercise also helps to get rid of vertigo.

Hair:

Is the crowning glory. Peel and chop one Spanish onion. Boil with a little water. Mix the juice with one teaspoon of castor oil and while hot rub into the scalp, gently massage and leave overnight – you may lose your partner but not your hair! Shampoo your hair in the usual way on the following morning. This remedy will not help those with a genetic hair loss disorder.

Bend your head forward and brush your hair away from your neck for one minute. This opens the pores of your scalp. Bending forward until your head faces the floor is a nourishment and stimulant to the hair follicles.

Head:

Carry your head splendidly and keep it still. There is no grace in a floundering head. Your ear lobs should be on a straight vertical line with your shoulder line. A twofold exercise: Lie on your back across the bed and let your head hang from the edge of the bed a few seconds every day. A sudden rush of blood to the head and face tones the tissues of the face and tightens the muscles under the chin.

Legs:

A stance: leg and foot position. Right foot should be slightly forward on which to place the greater weight of your body; and your left foot should be slightly behind with the foot and pad and firmly on the ground while the heel is raised a fraction; and your left knee slightly bent and touching the right knee.

Hands:

Rub your hands with one teaspoon honey mixed with quarter lemon juice, massaging well and rinse off. Alternative: the avocado/lemon juice preparation – see below. Get a pair of soft white gloves to wear at night at least once a week after application of hand treatment.

Ears:

Once a week put a drop or 2 of olive oil in each ear – prevents wax clogging the ears.

Nails:

Use emery paper rather than steel for nail care – at least once a week. Use cuticle fluid (home made) whenever you file your nails, apply around your nails and massage well; push the cuticles of your left fingers with your right thumb and vice versa. Then apply any of the above hand treatments, massaging well and rinse off. Once a week apply: dilute 1 teaspoon of coarse sea salt with 2 teaspoons of water; add 3 teaspoons of olive oil. Apply mixture to fingernails and toenails. This strengthens and enables them to grow.

Home made cuticle fluid -

Place in a jar one teaspoon of coarse sea salt (Palestinian, available from health shops); add two teaspoons of olive oil and use when required.

Facial make up:

For day care apply one layer of a light moisturiser such as pure avocado oil, olive oil, or a good brand of petroleum jelly to your face and when dry apply a sun cream for protection. If you prefer to use glamorous famous brands, be sure to remove make-up every night with a good deep cleansing cream followed by avocado treatment – lest your facial pores are in danger of clogging up, the agent of ageing facial skin.

Note: All the famous brands of glamorous make-up are based on petroleum jelly!

Stint and avoid caking up your face with make-up but don't stint your smile! Not only does a smile break the ice even with strangers but also exercises the tissues of your face.

The British Sun:

You need to be aware of two important things about the sun generally: Vitamin D deficiency, for lack of sun (VDD) and Sunstroke from excessive exposure to the sun.

Do not underestimate the power of the British sun! Author was born and raised in Africa where she suffered no sunstroke, but in Britain suffered two sun strokes: one in Scotland and another in England. There is a good number of people in Britain who suffer skin cancer caused by exposure to the sun; by underestimating the power of the British sun; and for lack of proper protective apparel or *sun creams*. Direct sun through window glass is particularly dangerous.

Lack of sunlight can cause VDD and the body suffers from extreme fatigue in some people and all sorts of unexplainable things may go wrong health wise. Diet alone may not help but the first thing is plenty of sunlight by spending much time in the sun, with appropriate protection, such as sun creams, sun glasses and a hat; and eating fortified foods.

Fortified food	Non fortified food
Cereal	Cod liver oil
Milk	Egg yolk
Orange juice	Canned: mackrell, salmon
Butter	(also farmed, wild & fresh),
	sardines, tuna, herrings (also fresh).

****

Prescribed drugs:

The human body is made up of different cells and this can be seen by the different ailments we suffer from; and for each a medical doctor will subscribe a drug or treatment for that particular ailment. In other words, one drug or treatment would not cure the whole body and may affect other parts of the body as side effects.

Yet, all the cells are inter-related and make up the whole body. We may look at cells as separate individuals each with its individual characteristics. Also note that every prescription obtained from the chemist is accompanied by an information sheet which suggests possible side effects to the drug among other things. The side effect(s) is a hostile reaction to the drug by some individual cells. Pay heed to the side effects and request an alternative to which the individual cells may be less hostile.

Avocado – multiple value:

Some say avocado is neither fruit nor vegetable, whatever it is, its properties are numerous and invaluable. Avocado is often avoided because of its high fat content. Consequently, its numerous benefits are overlooked. The oil extracted is widely used in the preparation of beauty products, such as creams, cleansers and moisturisers, to prevent the ageing effect of dehydration. It is also used in bath oils, shampoos, scalp conditioners and hair tonic. Avocado consumed together with other fruits and vegetables increases its value.

Blood Presure: the high potassium and folte content in avocado helps to regulate blood pressure, protects your body against circulatory diseases, heart problems and stroke. Cholesterol: Avocado contains oleic and linoleic acids that are effective in lowering the LDL cholesterol and increasing the healthy HDL cholesterol. **Bad Breath:** Avocado is among the best natural mouth wash and a remedy for bad breath; and it is effective in removing intestinal putrefactions which are the real cause of coated tongue. **Duodenal ulcer:** The blandness of avocado, as paw paw, is comforting and soothing to the hypersensitive surfaces of the stomach. **Eyesight:** The potent and anti-oxidant content in avocado helps neutralise free radicals that are vital for improving eyesight and prevents cataracts and glaucoma. **Fetal development:** the high folate content is important for healthy fetal cell and tissue development. **Immune system:** Regular consumption of avocados strengthens the body's immune system. **Kidney stones:** consumption of the high potassium content of avocado helps to reduce urinary calcium excretion, and lowers the risk of stones forming in the kidney. **Morning sickness:** The vitamin B6 in avocado relieves nausea associated with pregnancy. **Muscle and nerve:** the high potassium content in avocado helps balance the body's electolyes, acids muscle activity, nervefunction and energy metabolism.

Prostate cancer: certain phytpmitroemt content in avocado may help prevent the advancement of prostate cancer cells and may even help repair damaged cells.

****

Psoriasis: Psoriasis is an inherent psychological-related disorder, a kind of "skin-deep" parasite and does not scar the skin, though a condition in great need to focus on the *cause,* then follow the treatment. Psoriasis can appear through a variety of factors depending upon the circumstances of the patient; though it can also be genetic.

Living with psoriasis can be very uncomfortable. Psoris is also associated with osteoarthritis. Babies or young children who are not loved or do not receive enough or receive harsh attention, and where they have a fundamentally inherent psychological disorder may develop psoriasis. The writer noted that there were more cases of psoriasis suffered by women than by men, though this is by no means conclusive. Psoriasis can also be triggered by the apprehension of some imminent event, or the patient is bothered by some kind of *domination* of whatever nature in varying degrees.

The Facts

The facts are from the personal experience of the writer who has lived with psoriasis on and off since since 1986; and from research on the subject: Dr Andrew P Warin's video "A Touch of Psoriasis" and his CD-ROM "Switch on to Skin Problems"; general literature; and the observation of people who suffer from psoriasis.

The remedies studied and observed include *clothing*, *diet* and, particularly, *stressful situations*. brought about by a variety of factors.These factors may be deduced from the four examples offered out of the many cases the writer has explored and observed out of personal interest since 1986. Psoriasis can be a genetic or hereditary disease; hereditary in the sense that it is not the physical aspect of the anatomy of the patient that inherits the disorder; but rather the psychological aspect since the patient is psychologically unable to deal with the causes of stress for a number of reasons. Also present in those who suffer from psoriasis is the characteristic, in some instances, of the patient's own *defiant* nature towards an adverse situation.

Cases studied

A. Fear – Case of the author

Psoriasis was triggered by the apprehension of imminent death when the she was incarcerated in a small over-crowded prison cell on a space the size of a grave for five hours (and related circumstances, see book *From Blantyre to Blantyre*). Her ability to deal with stressful circumstances, even considerably trivial in comparison, became weakened. (Checking on ancestral history of psoriasis, only her great grandmother suffered from psoriasis).

B. Nagging – The director' wife

She was the wife of a retired director of a very large company. His job had been to lecture on various company methods to a very large number of personnel. A man of domineering nature, after retirement he could not get out of the habit of lecturing, rather turned to pontificating, by using his wife as an 'audience', (a nagging wife [so-called] situation reversed). He talked incessantly (except when he was asleep) and she could not get a word in on any subject. She failed to draw his attention to the fact that his incessant pontificating was getting her down.

The situation stressed her considerably and she could not deal with it, she could not leave him because of loyalty. In fluctuating degrees of seriousness she developed psoriasis.

C. Assertion – Mother's Boy

Mr C, an only child, lived with his mother and he never married. His mother dominated every aspect of his life and by her assertiveness she disap-proved of any of his friends, particularly female friends, and he was too weak to defy her. He suffered from psoriasis in varying degrees.

D. Bullying – The travel agent

Miss D worked as a travel agent in a large organisation. She was of a gentle nature and easily bullied by colleagues at the work place. She could not deal with the situation. Psoriasis set in.

Examples of the circumstances that cause stress abound. Suffice it to say that the person who develops psoriasis has, in the first place, a psychological genetic disorder, is bothered, irritated by *domination* of whatever nature and in varying degrees: the greater the bother the more serious the psoriasis. Because of a dominant factor, inability to retaliate, and/or loyalty the patient takes it out on herself or himself and reacts by scratching thereby aggravates the condition. Even though psoriasis may be eliminated by appropriate dermatological treatment, as soon as a stressful situation arises, even without the patient's knowledge, psoriasis may return with a vengeance.

Treatment for psoriasis

Topical Therapy

Whatever topical therapy is prescribed, emollients and salicylic acid (the various creams), is helpful and more comfortable to use at night: applied to the affected areas and covered with cling film, this also prevents staining slumber wear or bed linen; the scales are contained and can be disposed of by washing off or by having a bath or shower.

Intake of Steroids

The writer has found these to be unhelpful and the side effects to have a consequence of heat that has the tendency to cause itching and aggravates psoriasis. Avocado oil is helpful in the treatment of psoriasis, by applying twice a day to the affected areas. Avoid stressful situations. External and internal *heat* can escalate psoriasis, such as over-heated accommodation or temperatures that are irregular; clothing (particularly under garments); and diet. Sun heat is better than a cold climate, but with appropriate covering of clothing, such as a hat, sunglasses, etc. There is a tendency by some to wear too much clothing and this may aggravate psoriasis.

User hostile:	User friendly:
Central heating or storage heaters continuous hot temperature increases blood garments.	Silk: foundation garments, slumber wear, dressing gowns, blouses, and general
heat. Wool and too many	Lightweight cotton garments. layers of clothing.
Diet: alcohol, hot drinks, spices shell-fish, causes internal heat.	Gin-Seng, strong herbs Such as rosemary, and daily intake of detoxes. Yellow fruit, lettuce, and bananas.

Honey - a good cure for most ills:

Honey is the only food on the planet that will not spoil or rot. It will do what some call turning to sugar, but in reality honey is always honey. However, when left in a cool dark place for a long time it will do what I would rather call 'crystallise'. When this happens loosen the lid, boil some water, and sit the honey container in the hot water, turn off the heat and it will turn to liquid again. Never boil honey or put it in a microwave. To do so would kill the enzymes in the honey.

Honey is produced in most of the countries of the world. Scientists of today also accept honey as a medicine for all kinds of diseases. Honey can be used without any side effects for any kind of disease; if taken in the right dosage as a medicine, will not harm diabetic patients; and honey mixed with Cinnamon may cure most diseases (Weekly World News, 17/01/1995, Canadian magazine):

Mix 1 teaspoon honey with 1/4 teaspoon cinnamon powder and have at night for most cures.

Caution: Be sure you buy PURE honey. Most sellers today do not sell pure honey but mixed with all sort of things which should be avoided. It is best to buy honey from the health shop or directly from a local farm where the honey is produced.

Honey and Ginger for High Blood Pressure: Mix 1 table spoon of honey and 1 table spoon ginger (adrak) juice, 1 table spoon of crushed cumin seeds (jeera), and have it twice daily.

Heart Diseases: Honey and cinnamon powder, applied on bread, instead of jelly and jam, and eaten regularly for breakfast, will reduce cholesterol in the arteries and save one from heart attack. Those who have had a heart attack, if they do this process daily, they may keep next attack at bay; and this also relieves loss of breath and strengthens the heart beat.

Bladder Infections: To destroy germs in the bladder, take two tablespoons of cinnamon powder and one teaspoon of honey in a glass of lukewarm water.

Cholesterol: Two tablespoons of honey and three teaspoons of cinnamon powder mixed in 16 ounces of weak tea may reduce the level of cholesterol in the blood. Also pure honey taken with food reduces cholesterol.

Colds: One teaspoon honey and 1/4 teaspoon cinnamon powder in one tablespoon of lukewarm water taken daily for three days, may cure most chronic coughs, colds, and clear the sinuses.

Upset Stomach: Honey taken with cinnamon powder cures stomach ache and also clears stomach ulcers from the root.

Gas: According to the studies done in India and Japan, if Honey is taken with cinnamon powder the stomach is relieved of gas.

Immune System: Scientists have found that honey has various vitamins and iron in large amounts. Daily use of honey and cinnamon powder strengthens the immune system and protects the body from bacteria, and viral attacks; and strengthens the white blood corpuscles to fight bacterial and viral diseases.

Indigestion: Cinnamon powder sprinkled on two tablespoons of honey taken before food relieves acidity and digests the heaviest of meals. **Influenza:** A scientist in Spain proved that honey contains a natural 'ingredient' which kills the influenza germs and saves the patient from flu. **Longevity:** Tea taken regularly with honey and cinnamon powder, slows the ravages of old age: Four teaspoons of honey, one teaspoon of cinnamon powder, and three cups of water and boil together and drink ¼ three to four times a day. It keeps the skin fresh, soft and youthful.

Pimples: Apply a mixture of three tablespoons of honey and one teaspoon of cinnamon powder paste on the pimples before sleeping and wash off next morning with warm water. Pimples will be removed from the root if done daily for two weeks.

Skin Infections: In cases of eczema, ringworm and all types of skin infections, apply honey and cinnamon powder in equal parts on the affected areas of the body.

Weight Loss: On an empty stomach, daily in the morning one half hour before breakfast, and at night before sleeping, drink honey and cinnamon powder in one cup of boiling water. If taken regularly, it reduces the weight of even the most obese person. A regular intake of this mixture prevents fat from accumulating.

Cancer: Recent research in Japan and Australia revealed that advanced cancer of the stomach and bones have been cured successfully by taking daily one tablespoon of honey with one teaspoon of cinnamon powder for one month three times a day.

Fatigue: Recent studies have shown that the sugar content of honey is more helpful than detrimental to the strength of the body. The elderly, who take honey and cinnamon powder in equal parts, are more alert and supple. Half a tablespoon of honey taken in a glass of water and sprinkled with cinnamon powder, taken daily and about mid afternoon, when the energy of the body starts to decrease, after brushing teeth, increases the vitality of the body within a week.

Hearing Loss: Daily morning and night intake of equal parts of honey and cinnamon powder, restores hearing.

For those who seek natural remedies honey and cinnamon can also be taken in other ways for various things: a teaspoon of honey to a tablespoon of cyder vinegar, and ¼ teaspoon cinnamon in hot water when one has a cold; and for pollen allergies, a little honey and cinnamon will gradually build up immunity to pollen.

****

What We Eat

At age 45/50 aim to reduce intake of food and eat small portions frequently. Do not snack in between meals but drink a glass or two of water which helps to curb the appetite. For every meal use a small plate, measuring 9" diameter and a small bowl for breakfast.

Study your own body by trial and error while following your choice of recommended diet and pay heed to what you eat. There is much helpful literature on foods that harm and foods that heal. The first thing to remember is that food for others is poison for some. Regular activity will burn out the excess. Find an occupation, for boredom leads to comfort eating.

Virgin olive oil has multiple values, healthy heart and circulation but remember to use it in moderation for it can be rather fattening. Sprinkle olive oil to steamed hot vegetables, mix in salad dressing, if used for frying only thinly coat the pan – best to avoid fried foods altogether - use instead light tasting pure rapeseed oil or ground nut oil. Olive oil can also be used externally as a body moisturiser and to rub in your scalp before shampoo.

Olive oil, like avocado, are gentle oils to take internally and apply externally.

Allies

Avocados, almonds, most kinds beans, pulses, coconut milk, breast of chicken (no skin), courgettes, most fish: mackerel, salmon, sardine, tilapia, trout, molasses, wholemeal bread (anything with husk), whole wheat cereals, non-processed cheese, cottage cheese, sweet potatoes, cassava (manioc) yams, pasta, beans, pulses, squash, soy milk, low fat yoghurt, leafy vegetables, fresh fruit, broccoli, sunflower oil, whole eggs, all fresh fruit and vegetables, rice, millet, oats and pasta.

Note: If you suffer from a bowel disorder, avoid all beans and vegetables of the **Cruciferae** group (cabbage family): cabbage, broccoli, cauliflower, sprouts, kale, etc. Or anything that is gassy.

Good fat:

Polyunsaturated has several components but is not soaked with them. Omega 3: is found in oily fish such as salmon, mackerel, herring and trout; or oil in plants: walnut, rapeseed, soy beans and linseed.

Omega 6: Sunflower seeds, wheat germ, sesame, walnut, soy beans, corn and their oils, certain spreads but read the labels – see below.

Mono unsaturated – has solo component but is not soaked with it: olives, rapeseed and nuts: peanuts, pistachio, almonds, hazelnuts, macadamia, cashew and pecan, avocado and their oils.

Foes - Major foes: **salt, sugar and saturated fat**.

Salt: pre-prepared shop food already contains at least 75% of salt.

Sugar: most pre-prepared food also contains sugar.

If the packaging says 'SUGAR FREE' on it, LEAVE IT ALONE! It may contain Aspartame, which is considered dangerous: when the temperature of this sweetener exceeds 86 degrees F, the wood alcohol in ASPARTAME converts to formal aldehyde-alcohol, an oily colourless liquid by condensation of two

31

molecules of acetaldehyde and then to formic acid, which in turn causes metabolic acidosis. Formic acid is the poison found in the sting of fire ants. The methanol toxicity mimics, among other conditions, multiple sclerosis and systemic lupus.

Fat: for a healthy heart eating beware of foods that have hidden fat:

Saturated: bread, cakes, cheese, butter, full fat milk and yoghurt, pies,biscuits, pastries, lard, dripping, hard margarine and baking fat, coconut and palm oil, meat and meat products such as sausages or hamburgers.

Avoid: White bread, white sugar, biscuits, chocolates, save above but not minimum 70% cocoa, sweets, doughnuts, hamburgers, processed meats or cheese, smoked meals or fish, margarine, animal fat, stale food, citrus, pizza, saturated fat, cow's milk and cream, heavy spices, fried foods, tinned food, cheap wine, excessive alcohol, processed soy products, as most processed foods and pastry, burnt food or burnt toast.

Trans fat: Frying and baking fat, such as hydrogenated vegetable oils used in biscuits, cakes and pastries, dairy products, animal fat such as beef, lamb, pork and chicken fat, particularly chicken skin. Fast foods contain much of trans fat.

Food labels: when you purchase food you should look out for the labels which indicate the content of the item. Labels come in red, Amber and Green. Red is high; amber is medium and green is low.

Examples:

Per 100g	**Too much is:**	**Less is:**
Total fat	20g	3g
Saturated fat	5g	1g
Salt (sodium)	1.5g (0.5g)	3g (0.1g)
Sugar	10g per 100g	2g per 100g

The Red represents foods we should try to cut down on or avoid completely. Amber is better most of the time and green is the best healthy choice. If some reds are foods you like strive to consume very little only. Gassy foods tend to blow up your abdomen, such as the Cruciferae family, legumes, onions, particularly Spanish, peppers, citrus and fizzy drinks.

Avoid: lack of fluid or sleep, stress, alcohol, caffeine, hot cocoa, acidic fruit juices. In air travel take fluids, preferably water, as one tends to become dehydrated beginning from a certain level in the air.

Allies – in moderation:

Carbohydrates: Bread, rice, corn, millet, pasta, cereal, potatoes, whole grain bread, rolls and tortillas and whole wheat pita, fresh fruit, fresh vegetables, raisins, potatoes, sweet potatoes and bananas. Protein: Meat, fish, eggs, cheese, milk, tofu, edamame (steamed soya rejuvenated beans), fresh soya beans, yoghurt, lean chicken, fish, egg whites and avocado. **Nutrients:** carbohydrates, vitamins, minerals, fat (energy). Your body needs fat but choose the right kind.

Calories: choose low fat.

Vitamins	What it improves	Intake
A	eyesight	liver, butter, cheese, milk,
	brain	cereals, yeast, wheat germ.
B	Anti-oxidants	carrots & tomatoes
B1	appetite (thiamine)	liver, kidney, milk, green bilberry, colts foot, cranberry, and dong quai.
B2	hair growth	vegetables and mushrooms.
	Alertness	
B12	Energy	liver, kidney, red meat, eggs,
	Cholesterol	and dairy products in moderation.
BBC	Oestrogen	tofu, almond milk, broccoli greens, fish, vegetables, raw food and fresh fruit juice.
	Calcium	
C	Cartilage	citrus, currants, berries, melons, lettuce, peppers, beans, sprouts, raw cabbage, kiwi, melon and strawberries.
	Colds	
D	Bones, teeth	Sunlight, animal fat, eggs, butter (moderate) tuna, herrings, sardine.
	Suppleness	
E	Sex gland	vegetable oils, maize oil, fresh soya beans, yams, sweet potato, peanut

	Hormone	and coconut.
K	Blood	kale, spinach, all greens, milk, cheese, yoghurt, whole grain, cereals, red meat, offal, sardines, beans, peas, berries, barley, whole grain cereals.
	Calcium	
	Iron	

Antioxidant	Blueberries.

Herbs

Herbs are very important as one form of aiding youthfulness. Drink them, eat them and add them to food cooked or raw. Contact the herbalist for advice and supply and take them sensibly - they are an essential part of diet.

Diuretic	**Antibiotic**	**Anaemia and skin**
Alfafa	Garlic	Nettle
Cranberry	Ginger	Parsley
Dandelion	Fennel	Apricots
	Oregano	Spnach
	Sarsaparilla	

Eyes/vascular	Digestive	Psoriasis
Bilberry	Cabbage	Aloe Vera (external)
Cheese	Currants	Black walnut
Carrots	Kiwi	Burdock
Eye bright	Lettuce	Nettle
Liver	Melon	Sarsaparilla
Milk	Peppers	Fennel
	Sprouts	Cucumber
	Ginger	

Allergies	Sinuses	Colds & cholesterol
Cereals	Beans	Colts foot
Greens	Grain	Echiana
Liquorice	Eye bright	Garlic
Mushrooms	Eggs, whole	Horseradish
Nettle	Horseradish	Lemon balm
Wheat germ	Marshmallow	Onions, oats.

Hair & Calcium	Blood cleanser	Blood pressure and
Horsetail	and thinning	Palpitations
Dandelion	Hawthorn berry	Garlic, Parsley

Coughs &	Fatigue	Alertness
Lung congestion	Borage, Ginseng	Ginkgo
Garlic, Liquorice	Gotu Kola	Gotu Kola
Peppermint	Liquorice	
Breath	Anti-fungal	Liver
Calendula	Black walnut	Milk thistle
Peppermint	Pau D'Arco	
White oak bark	Slippery elm	
Cinnamon		

Fever	Gums	Cramps
Lemon balm	Red raspberry	Valerian
Energy	A teaspoon of honey on a cream cracker	
Apple	will also give you instant energy – natural	
Celery	sweetness is better than binging on	
Ginger, fresh	confectionery.	
Kiwi		

To Reduce Weight – follow options 1 and 2 for at least 2-4 weeks. Do not starve to slim but keep a regular routine of meal times and avoid nibbling in between meals. Fill yourself up with vegetables, no overcooking and no carbohydrates:

Option 1 - Green soy beans, leeks, green beans, peas, leafy vegetables, carrots, parsnips and herbs (raw and chopped), add half cup water and boil on high heat for 5 minutes with lid on.

Switch off and leave to steam for 10 minutes. Serve with a sprinkling of extra virgin olive oil and small quantify of protein of choice: chicken, fish, lamb or cottage cheese.

Option 2 - Carrots, parsnips, mixed sweet peppers, courgette, turnips or swede, sweet potatoes and herbs; and sprinkle a few drops of sunflower/vegetable oil and one cup of water. Roast in oven for 20 minutes. Serve with protein of choice. Do not use olive oil, as cooked olive oil loses its value.

1 **Always eat slowly**
2 **Focus on:**
>   Cinnamon which lowers blood sugar/cholesterol.
>   Ginger
>   Beats nausea – preserve fresh ginger in dry sherry
>   in fridge.
>   Basil
>   Combats stress.

Mono unsaturated fatty acid:

>   1.OILS – Canola, sesame, soy bean, walnut, flaxseed,
>   sunflower, olive, and peanut.
>   2.OLIVES – source of iron, Vit E, copper, fibre
>   3.NUTS & SEEDS – sunflower seed, Pistachios
>   4.AVOCADOS – packed with lutein, flavanols
>   5.DARK CHOCOLATE, not below 70% cocoa.

Categories of calories you burn:

>   1.Basal   - energy cells used to perform daily muscle
>   contractions

2.Activity - exercise, whatever.
3.Digestion – food.

Bloating of tummy may be caused by: lack of fluid; stress; lack of sleep; in air travel (take fluids); and avoid Alcohol, coffee, tea, hot cocoa, acidic fruit juices; and the cruciferous vegetable of the family Brassicaceae (also called Cruciferae: cabbage, garden cress, bok choy, broccoli, brussels sprouts and similar green leaf vegetables).

Avoid the following:

1. **Excess carbs**: pasta, banana, bagels, pretzels
2. **Bulky raw foods:** uncooked carrots.
3. **Gassy foods**: legumes, Cruciferae group, onions, peppers, citrus.
4. **Chewing gum**
5. **Sugar alcohols: cookies, candy, energy bars.**
6. **Fried foods**
7. **Spicy foods**, black pepper, nutmeg, cloves, chilli, hot sauces, malt vinegar, garlic, and mustard.
8. **Carbonated** drinks, fizzy drinks.

Routine - Daily basics:

Eat fresh food every day and do not keep food beyond 24 hours. This means do not prepare more than you need.

Breakfast options:

1 or 2 tablespoons organic porridge oats, soak in ½ or 1 cup hot water for 5 minutes, cook on low heat for five minutes. Add 1 tablespoon of low fat natural yoghurt and half teaspoon honey.

1 tablespoon muesli, soak in 1 cup hot water for 5 minutes. Add 1 tablespoon of low fat natural yoghurt – see muesli recipe

below.

1 tablespoon oatmeal soak in 1 cup boiling water for 5 minutes, cook on low heat for 10 minutes. Add 1 tablespoon natural low fat yoghurt and half teaspoon honey.

Elevenses

Drink a glass of water, decaffeinated tea or decaffeinated coffee or unsweetened fruit juice. Eat choice of slice of Cindy cake – see recipe below; or a cracker or two spread with half teaspoon of honey; or two/three dates or a mixture of dried fruit and nuts; or Fruit bar – see recipe below; or Fruit salad: In a small bowl, place peeled chopped mango, paw paw, apricots, grapes, kiwi, banana or melon. Yellow fruit is good for the skin. Best buy is dried apricots from a health shop, sugar-free: soak a few in cold water and keep in fridge.

Lunch options – to fit a 9" diameter plate – do not pile up lest you lose the purpose of a small plate:

Salad: Fresh apple slithers or grated, grated cucumber, rocket or lettuce leaves – if you do not suffer from arthritis add tomatoes – then include a choice of a few slices of avocado, or tinned sardines, or prawns, or cottage cheese or boiled egg. Eat with cream crackers or crisp bread or bread made from soy flour.

Afternoon refreshment - choice of any one of the Elevenses or lemonade - see recipes below.

Dinner 6pm: main meal - since you have no way of burning excessive calories at night. You may wish to transpose the main meal and have it at mid-day if that suits you.

Recipes - Salt is optional in all the following dishes.

Salad cream:

Make in a bowl a paste of 2 teaspoons of corn flour and a teaspoon of cold milk, pour over 1 cup of hot milk stirring all the time, place all in a saucepan and cook thoroughly on low heat.

When cool add:

> 2 teaspoons olive oil)
>
> 2 teaspoons Balsamic white vinegar) Liquidise all in
>
> 1 teaspoon English mustard) a blender
>
> 1 boiled free range egg yolk)
>
> 2 teaspoons fresh cream)
>
> Capers, salt and pepper to taste)

Keep in fridge and use within 4 days. The taste of some dishes is improved by blending in a liquidiser. To the above add sweet pepper purée as a dressing for prawns.

Sweet pepper purée:

2 large red sweet peppers – chop and put in liquidiser with a little water, place in small containers and keep in freezer. Use when required, for no more than 1 week.

Sweet pepper garnish – for flavouring and colour:

> 4 large sweet peppers, red, orange and green
>
> remove seeds and chop fine.
>
> In 1 tablespoon hot rapeseed oil sauté 3 chopped spring onions,

on high heat for three minutes;

add fresh garlic paste, herbs, cook for 2 minutes;

add peppers, and 3-minute pre-steamed, *petit pois* (peas),

stir fry for 3 minutes.

Remove from cooker without lid to keep dry.

When cool freeze in small containers and use when required.

Chicken -

Breast:

Recipe 1: Slice breast lengthwise, do not separate, fill with mixture of:

> 1 tablespoon of sage and onion filling;
> 1 teaspoon soy spread;
> ¼ teaspoon garlic paste;
> 2 teaspoons coconut milk; and
> 1 tablespoon boiling water.

Lightly coat pan with rapeseed oil, place prepared chicken and cover with whole mange tout or frozen green beans, steam on lowest heat mark for five minutes with lid on. Turn over and steam for 3 minutes.

Before serving cut into 2" slices.

Chicken schnitzel (Polish):

Cut into 4 or more pieces of chicken breast. Beat with a wooded meat tenderizer, place in a bowl and add: finely chopped herbs, garlic paste, two tablespoons coconut milk, and one teaspoon paprika; mix well and coat with breadcrumbs. Sparsely cover frying pan with rapeseed oil, on medium heat; when hot sauté the chicken pieces – they brown very quickly. Serve with ziemniaki (bashed potatoes, see recipe below) and vegetables.

By courtesy of Izabela Brzezinska, Manchester, England.

Chicken paprika:

Pieces of chicken on the bone (no breast) and marinate with:

    1 tablespoon paprika (chilli powder optional)
    Mix well and leave
    1 teaspoon garlic paste ....) overnight, then
    1 tablespoon coconut milk....) grill.
    Chopped fresh herbs ....)

Polish recipe for ziemniaki (potatoes):

Prepare potatoes, well cover in pan of cold water with half teaspoon salt. When cooked drain off all the water. Replace pan with lid on switch off cooker for a few seconds, remove, hold tight and vigorously shake the pan.

By courtesy of Magdalena Staniszewska, Bolton England.

Fish:

Use a saucepan especially for cooking fish and do not use it for anything else, lest you spoil the taste of other foods. Choose oil rich fish such as salmon, sardine, trout, pilchards, bloaters, whitebait, mackerel, herring, kippers, sprats or brisling which help to protect the heart. Line a saucepan with chopped spring onions, garlic paste, fresh chopped herbs and place fish on top, cover with a few leafy vegetables. Cook on high heat for 3 minutes, and steam for 10 minutes on lowest heat with lid on.

Rice and peppers:

To 1 cup of Basmati rice (if using other brands be sure to drain off water before steaming) add one and half cup boiling water and one tablespoon coconut milk, and whole cinnamon bark. Cook on high heat for 3 minutes, reduce heat to lowest mark and cook with lid on until water dries off – 3-5 minutes. Switch off cooker and steam for 3 minutes. Mix in sweet pepper garnish. Serves 4.

Green mango chutney:

2 lbs sliced green mangoes)

Place all in large saucepan, add malt

2 chopped shallot onions   )   vinegar to cover, about 2 pints
and

4 cloves garlic, cut in half) 1 cup water. Bring to boil,

reduce heat to

Half cup sultanas   )   lowest mark and cook

slowly till moisture

Half cup peanuts   ) is almost dry. When cool place

in jars

2 peeled and sliced apples) with lids tightly on.

1 teaspoon each of salt,   )

Cinnamon, mixed spice,   )

1 lb soft brown sugar   )

Chillie powder optional   )

Source: Nyasaland (Malawi) Council of Women (British) *Cookery Book*

and Household Guide, 1947.

Deserts:

You can't leave me alone – queen of desserts:

2 eggs – whisk yolks with 2 tablespoons of caster sugar.

Add: juice of 2 lemons; and 2 tablespoons gelatine,

dissolved in half cup hot water.

Whisk the egg whites very stiff and fold in. Put in glass bowl and place in the fridge until set. Add a layer of raspberry jam and cover with whipped cream.
Source: Nyasaland Council of Women (British) *Cookery Book and*

Household Guide, 1947.

Ice Cream Dream:

Mix 450g of any frozen berries; 2 egg whites; 225g caster sugar and mix in a food processor. Whip 240ml double cream, 2 teaspoons vanilla essence, 2 egg yolks and mix. Stir all ingredients together and freeze.

By courtesy of Helen Spencer, Bolton, England.

Cindy cake – no fat, no sugar:

2 cups mixed fruit: raisins, sultanas, chopped) Put all in a bowl

dates, 1 teaspoon each of cinnamon and   ) add 2 mugs cold
tea

mixed spice   ) and leave overnight.

Add: 1 cup oat meal   ) Mix well, pour in greased
square

2 cups porridge oats   ) baking tin "18 x12" and bake in

2 teaspoons baking powder   ) pre-heated oven.

3 beaten eggs

Cool, cut into 6 squares and place in fridge or in freezer. Use
within two weeks.

NOTE: Sugar-free dried fruit can be found in health shops.

Snack bars:

1 cup porridge oats, half cup each of:) Mix together and pour
in

Oat bran, wheat germ, dried chopped) greased square tin
17"x12".

fruit, sugar-free from health shop;   ) and bake in pre-
heated oven.

4 oz. Soy or sunflower spread   )

1 cup sesame seeds; and   ) When cool turn out and

1 cup hot water.   cut into slices.

Muesli:

3 cups plain, unsweetened oat muesli) Mix and place in a

½ cup mixed dried fruit- sugar-free.   ) container and use

2 tablespoons wheat germ   ) when required.

½ cup mixed seeds   )

Lettuce soup – a relaxing soup

4 leaves of lettuce   ) Boil together for 10

1 medium size potato, peeled   ) minutes and leave

cut in two, and 1 cup water   ) to cool.

Liquidise and pour in saucepan with 1 cup milk and heat for

4 minutes, add salt and pepper to taste. Serve with a lacing of fresh cream on top.

Thousand Vegetable soup – a dependable basic:

Chop: carrot, spring onion, courgette, mange tout, add 2 tablespoons frozen peas and green beans - add or use as many vegetables as you wish, the more the better.

Place 1 tablespoon soy spread and sauté all together in a saucepan for 3 minutes. Add one cup of water and cook for 10 minutes on lowest heat; when cool liquidise and replace to saucepan with water, salt and pepper to taste.

Butternut soup – queen of soups:

Boil one half of butternut, when cool scoop out. Peel and grate half a Spanish onion, 1 clove garlic and sauté in one tablespoon of rapeseed oil or soy spread.

Add 1 and one half cups milk and mix well with the butternut.

Add salt and pepper to taste and one tablespoon of fresh cream before serving.

By courtesy of Mary Marne, Blantyre Malawi.

Lemonade:

Add 200g sugar to the zest and juice of 6 lemons and 2 limes.

Add one and one half litres hot water and stir. Cover, cool and chill.

By courtesy of Helen Spencer, Bolton, England.

Meat:

No meat recipes are offered in this booklet. Meat protein is difficult to digest, requires a lot of digestive enzymes, and becomes putrefied leading to more toxic build-up in the stomach. Water alone will not detox the problem and you may have to take an anti-biotic herb – see under Herbs or seek medical help. Meat feeds cancer cells.

Light supper:

Have a light supper between 9:00-10:00 pm of vegetable soup or a cracker with a hot drink or half a banana which is also relaxing - so you do not feel hungry or get indigestion from lack of food at night.

Spice for cure –

The people of India originally used spices to cure certain ills and gradually began to add them into their cooking. The author loves spices but they are hostile to her. Therefore, no spicy recipes have been offered. Bisides the Asian shops, one can now purchase spice items, at most supermarkets.

Ajwain/Ajmo for Asthma:

Boil ajwain in water and inhale the steam. Arthritis: Turmeric helps to avoid arthritis and most problems. It contains anti-inflammatory property and it can be taken as a drink other than adding to dishes. To one teaspoon of turmeric powder add a cup of warm milk every day. Bitter Gourd/Karela: A tablespoon of amla juice mixed with a cup of fresh bitter gourd (karela) juice and taken daily for 2 months reduces blood sugar. Blocked Nose.For blocked nose or to relieve congestion, take a table spoon of crushed carom seeds (ajwain), tie it in a cloth and inhale. Colds: Mix a gram of cinnamon powder with a teaspoon of honey to cure a cold. Prepare a cup of tea to which you should add ginger, clove, bay leaf and black pepper. This should be consumed twice a day. Reduce the intake as the cold disappears. Cramps: A self-massage with mustard oil every morning helps cramps. Just take a little oil between your palms and rub it all over your body. Then take a shower. This is especially beneficial during winter. You could also mix a little mustard powder with water to make a paste and apply this on your palms and soles of your feet. Backache: Rub ginger paste on the backache to get relief. Dry Cough: Add a gram of turmeric powder to a teaspoon of honey for curing a dry cough. Also chew a cardamom for a long time. Garlic for High Blood Pressure: Have 1-2 pod garlic first thing in the morning with water. Ginger for Colds: Ginger tea is very good to cure a cold: cut ginger into small pieces and boil it with water, for a few times and then add honey to sweeten or milk to taste, and drink while hot. Heart: Turmeric lowers cholesterol and by preventing the formation of the internal blood clots improves circulation and prevents heart disease and stroke. Turmeric canbe taken as a drink other than adding to dishes to help prevent most problems. Use one teaspoon of turmeric powder per cup of warm milk every day.

Indigestion: Turmeric can be used to relieve digestive problems like ulcers, dysentery, and can be taken as a drink to help prevent most problems. Use one teaspoon of turmeric powder per one cup of warm milk every day. **Headaches:** If you have a regular migraine problem, include five almonds along with hot milk in your daily diet. You could also have a gram of black pepper along with honey or milk, twice or thrice a day. Make an almond paste by rubbing wet almonds against a stone. This can be applied to the forehead. Eat an apple with a little salt on an empty stomach every day and see its wonderful effects. When headache is caused by cold winds,cinnamon works best in curing headache. Make a paste of cinnamon by mixing in water and apply it all over your forehead. **Hiccups:** Take a warm slice of lemon and sprinkle salt, sugar and black pepper on it. The lemon should be eaten until the hiccups stop. **High Blood/Cholesterol:** In 1 glass of water, add 2 tablespoons of coriander seeds and bring to boil. Let the concoction cool for some time, strain, and drink the mixture twice a day. Or Sunflower seeds, which are extremely beneficial, as they contain linoleic acid that helps to reduce the cholesterol deposits on the walls of arteries.

High Blood Pressure: Have 1-2 pod garlic (lasan) first thing in the morning with water. Or mix 1 tablespoon honey and 1 tablespoon ginger juice, 1 table spoon of crushed cumin seeds and have it twice daily. It also works as an ntiseptic for injuries. **Migraine:** For the cure of migraine or acute cold in the head; boil a tablespoon of ground pepper, and a pinch of turmeric in a cup of milk, and have it daily for a few days. Best cure for persistent migraine is to avoid groups of food such as all dairy; or all citrus, by trial and error. **Piles:**

Radish juice should be taken twice a day, once in the morning and then later in the night. Initially drink half a of cup of radish juice and then gradually increase it to a full cup; or soak 3-4 figs in a glass of water and keep overnight. Eat the figs on an empty stomach, the next morning. **Sinusitis:** Mango serves as an effective home remedy for preventing the frequent attacks of sinus, and mango contains much of vitamin A. Alternatively, add raw onion and garlic in your daily meals. Or Fenugreek leaves are considered valuable in curing sinusitis. In 250 ml water, boil 1 teaspoon of Fenugreek seeds, till reduced to half, then inhale. This will help you to perspire, dispel toxicity and reduce fever. Or tie a teaspoon of black cumin seeds in a thin cotton cloth and inhale. **Sore Throat:** Add a teaspoon of cumin seeds and a few small pieces of dry ginger to a glass of boiling water. Simmer it for a few minutes, and then let it cool. Drink it twice daily. This will cure a cold as well as sore throat. **Tonsillitis:** Take a fresh lemon and squeeze it in a glass of water. Add 4 teaspoons of honey and one teaspoon of salt; and drink it slowly sip by sip. Also milk has proved beneficial in treating tonsillitis. In 1 glass of pure boiled milk, add a pinch of turmeric powder and ground pepper and drink it every night for about 3 days. **Turmeric/Arad cure for injuries:** For any cut or wound, apply turmeric powder to the injured portion to stop the bleeding. It also works as an antiseptic. You can tie a bandage after applying turmeric. **Urinary Tract Infection:** In 8 oz of water, put 1 teaspoon of baking soda and drink it, and drink plenty of cold water, as it aids in flushing out the waste products from the body. Or drink Cranberry juice. You can also add some apple juice for taste. **Vomiting:** Take 2 cardamoms and roast them on a dry pan. Grind the cardamoms, add a teaspoon of honey. Drink this frequently. It serves as a home remedy for vomiting. Alternatively, in a mixture of 1 teaspoon of mint juice and 1 teaspoon lime juice, add 1 teaspoon of ginger juice and 1 teaspoon honey; and drink the mixture. Or take a glass of chilled lime juice and sip slowly. Alternatively, drink ginger tea; or in a glass water, add some honey and drink, sip by sip. **Warts:** Apply castor oil daily over the warts and continue for several months. Or apply milky juice of fresh and barely-ripe figs a number of times a day for two weeks. Or rub cut raw potatoes on the affected area several times daily. Continue for at least two weeks. Alternatives to this is to apply on the warts: peeled and sliced onions to stimulate the circulation of blood; milk from the cut end of a dandelion 2-3 times a day; oil extracted from the shell of the cashew nut; papaya juice; or pineapple juice.

What We Drink

It is better not to drink cheap wine at all. British wines are good but some people are hooked on particularly French labels. A change of attitude from French labels came with the emergence on the market of South African and Australian wines. Wine and alcohol in general, will always remain the choice of the individual. The key is to consume as little alcohol as possible, excessive drinking can lead to many problems: one is alcohol dependency and the effect it has to health in general and to the mind. For some, alcohol can aid fast ageing, while to others it does not affect them at all, no matter how much they drink.

****

What We Do

Clubs:

Look for and join a club that involves activity, the major aim is to keep active but also enjoying what you are doing: Cycling,

Dance, Golf, Horse riding, Swimming (author has never been able to conquer fear of water and has had many beautiful swimsuits that never got wet!), T'ai Chi, Walking, Yoga, or any other activity that might suit you – to achieve near perfect athletic condition.

You may find a companion less oppressed or depressed than yourself in activity clubs. Some clubs established, supposedly for the purpose of combating loneliness of the singles, seldom provide the services advertised. Some managers of singles clubs do well lucratively from annual dues; and others con lonely hearts - beware. Nonetheless, a good number of such clubs provide the services they advertise and if one can find such a club it is a worthwhile pastime.

Once at a singles club, women resorted to dancing with other women in the favourite tune: "I will survive [without him]". Men grouped themselves together holding the supportive pint discoursing on the shortcomings of past relationships (instead of putting such things behind them). Unless one hasbeen formally introduced, approach by self-introduction may be regarded as 'pushy' - the English social syndrome. As a consequence, England has the greatest number of lonely men and women in Britain, according to author's observation.

Rest and exercise:

Both rest and exercise are essential to good health and renewed energy.

Rest: As we grow older we tend to sleep less, for most about four or five hours a night, consequently the day is longer to cope with. Take a daily siesta for a couple of hours even if you may fall asleep for only less than an hour. Even a ten-minute sleep can charge up your energy. It was Winston Churchill's daily ten-minute nap that won the Second World War - other things considered of course! He completely shut off the troubles of war in those ten minutes to awaken to renewed energy and think up his war strategy.

Exercise:

A well exercised body is a fit one and exercise can come in many forms, the key is activity. A sedentary existence is an enemy of the human body. Visit your local gym at least twice a week. Most gym personnel are well-trained and very helpful in advising what is best for you.

Or if you are inclined to gardening and are physically able, grow your own organic vegetables. Also do simple exercises at home. Put on your favourite dance music and dance around the house while doing your chores.

Take a positive attitude to your household chores and regard them as a form of therapy - while you are still able to do so, for a time will come when your body will simply refuse to do any chore. Try to do all the cleaning yourself but do not attempt to clean the windows or climb on house ladders to do chores, especially if you suffer from vertigo lest you trip and fall.

****

What We Think

What we think is an *attitude of mind* which in one sense has not entirely been a personal choice because we live in a system of 'coded categories' and one of them is *Ageism*. Statutory requirement enforced retirement at a certain age and though not any more since 1 October 2011, it would take time for this situation to become adjusted and jobs may not always be available for those who wish to continue working.In any event, the way around this is to *refuse to retire* – a retired attitude is the road to progressive ageing. Where it is not possible to find a placement there are many in our beautiful world in need of the most basic things of daily existence and charity institutions always welcome volunteer workers. It is not always best to say "what's in it for me" – it is by giving that we receive.

An alternative is to establish a small personal business if one is that way inclined. There is much useful information on the internet on self-employment – though some advise is for sale – or a local office where such information can be obtained. The local Age UK or the local Citizens Advice Bureau may direct one to the appropriate organisation in a variety of subjects besides self-employment.

****

Dress Code:

Celebrate the season by selecting trendy outfits but suitable for you. Strive to avoid the 'mutton dressed like lamb' look. Don't worry if you do not have the Joy Adams legs for mini skirts, wear what pleases you but sometimes aim to leave something to the imagination. Mix and match separate garments while paying attention to colour blending: grey, purple and pink; black, white and red; blue, green and red; navy and white. Try not to blend more than three colours for a single outfit. Follow the same pattern for your accessories.

According to reflexologists, when you wear high heel shoes you are literally walking on your forehead. The foot is a replica of your entire body. High heels will damage your feet. Consider orthopaedic bespoke (specially made for you) shoes – it is better to have one or two pairs of quality shoes than many pairs that hurt and not suitable for your feet.

Choose a sling bag – preferably small – rather than the handbag and try to carry as little as you can. Avoid carrying everything in your bag – travel light as it helps your posture.

Mirror:

It is said "A woman will never cease to look on the bright side of the mirror" – though some men monopolise the mirror! Have a full length mirror and most importantly when you look into the mirror stand sideways, you will then be able to check your posture, back and tummy.

It is also great fun to have your own private fashion parade and ask a friend or friends what they think about your outfits. The view of another can be more helpful than your own assessment on the suitability for you.

Take a few minutes exercise indoors by walking while holding a stick across your back or play a 'dance tune' and dance around – it helps to avoid the 'dowager hump' and improves your posture.

Books and useful information:

Bates Brothers, Greengrocers

C4 Ashburner Street, Bolton Market.

Fresh exotic fruit, vegetables and herbs.

John Hool Herbalist

C4 Ashburner Street, Bolton Market.

Advice on herbs.

Tel: 01204 391663 – www.herbalist-online.com

The Doctors Book of Home Remedies for Women

By the Editors of *Prevention* Magazine Health Book

Rodel Press Inc. Emmans, Pennsylvania, USA

Margaret Hills, Treating Arthritis the Drug-Free Way

SRN. New edition revised by Christine Horner, ECNP,

MRNT. ISBN 978-1-84709-005-8.

Joan Collins, *Looking Good, Feeling Great,*

Robson Books, 64 Brewery Road, London N7 9NT

QUOTATIONS –

An intelligent enemy is less dangerous than a foolish friend.

An organisation is reflected by the calibre of its personnel.

A positively focused mental attitude is more likely to achieve success.

A rock is dependable but not a stone.

Assert your rights and be firm in your belief.

A thief is a thief only when caught.

Be in good terms with all people and things.

Belonging is the key to living.

Cliques are the norm of existence.

Do not impose yourself where you are not welcome.

Every conception, every birth, is a winner but we are blinkered

by cussedness.

Fashion is cruel and it kills individualism.

Good counsel is concealed in a bad situation.

Handsome is s/he who exudes kindness.

Keeping up with the achievers is the road to want.

Know all, say all is verbal diarrhea.

Love, truth, peace, and charity are indestructible qualities.

Never argue with a fool they may not know the difference.

No one gets to the top without the help of others.

No one is responsible for one's failures but one self.

Rudeness is a silent killer.

Self-denigration is a psychological malady but cancer is a biological and psychological disorder.

Speak your truth calmly and quietly.

The basis of true happiness is good thoughts.

The boss's eye is God's own presence.

The limbs of body are the sword of the mind.

The body cannot miss what the mind has not perceived – Cave dwellers were content in their existence.

The best way to beat them is by the law of their land or by their own stick.

The consequences of omission are as grave as the consequences of commission.

The most important things are invisible, as truth or love.

To dwell upon yesterday's folly is to miss living today.

To harbour a grievance is to walk alone.

To walk on those who are down is an act of cruelty.

Waste is the road to want.

Weather and climate determine fashion.

Where logic ends the political reality begins.

****

Youth

It is a benefit to set aside experience and thank heaven for the Youth – how could we cope in a modern world? It is their world, they are well conversant with it and all the modern technology that goes with it – we can learn so much from them – some of their youth may even rub off on us!

****

EPILOGUE

The human body is a thing of beauty and the soul within is of ultimate beauty. The body is made up of trillions of cells and each cell has its own characteristics, of long or short span of life. This is why we get disorders in different parts of the body as seen by the doctor's prescription for that particular ailment. The body is a tabernacle or God's temple that houses the soul during its temporal sojourn through earth - body should be treated with respect and care. 1 Corinthians, 3:16:

"Don't you know that you yourselves are God's temple and

that God's Spirit dwells in your midst?"

From the author's experience, selective diet can offer practical solutions to good health. The right nutrition can prevent and treat a good number of diseases, though modern medicine is never prepared to accept this...and the wrong diet can attack the weak cells, in some instances leading to premature death.

The author does not claim to offer a panacea for eternal youth, subjected as we are to the natural laws of evolution from conception and beyond death motivated by linear time. It is possible to harness a good quality of life, good health and well being by food, fluid, thought, lifestyle and exercise which are vital to the maintenance of a healthy mind and body and youthfulness. Youth is within us as is the fountain of love in our bosom. One does not seek the impossible, the human body was not made to last forever, but to improve the quality of life –

where there is life there is hope.

****

Parting Thought

The Dining Table:

Respect the dining table and avoid in-between snacking on junk food in public - there is time and place for everything. Share the day's experiences and anecdotes at the end of a day with your family, the fundamental rock of your life, regardless of the type of family you belong to: two parents, single parent whether within or without wedlock, heterosexual, lesbian or gay – you were not responsible for the circumstances of your conception or for the care received in tender years.

In adulthood weed out certain aspects of your childhood conditioning and find your own identity:

> You are as good as anyone –
>
> No one is better than you –
>
> You are no better than anyone –

This little booklet is packed with information on how to harness good health and a youthful existence, based upon the lifestyle we lead. Aimed to aid the body and mind in what to do in our daily lives, the author discusses the importance of herbs, their uses and qualities... guidance particularly in advancing age... and for anyone who is keen to maintain vitality in a youthful existence.

www.ingramcontent.com/pod-product-compliance
Lightning Source LLC
Chambersburg PA
CBHW052107270326
41931CB00012B/2918